MS
c.)

FLR $17.95 c.)

Lyme Disease

By Judy Monroe

Perspectives on Disease and Illness

LifeMatters
an imprint of Capstone Press
Mankato, Minnesota

LifeMatters Books are published by Capstone Press
PO Box 669 • 151 Good Counsel Drive • Mankato, Minnesota 56002
http://www.capstone-press.com

©2001 Capstone Press. All rights reserved. No part of this book may be reproduced or transmitted in any form or by any means without written permission from the publisher. The publisher takes no responsibility for the use of any of the materials or methods described in this book nor for the products thereof.

Printed in the United States of America

Library of Congress Cataloging-in-Publication Data
Monroe, Judy.
    Lyme disease / by Judy Monroe.
        p.   cm. — (Perspectives on disease and illness)
    Includes bibliographical references and index
    ISBN 0-7368-0751-9
    1. Lyme disease—Juvenile literature. [1. Lyme disease. 2. Diseases.] I. Title. II. Series.
    RC155.5 .M66 2001
    616.9´2—dc21   00-030187
                                                                                  CIP

    Summary: Explains what Lyme disease is, what its symptoms are, and how it is spread. Also describes ways to avoid Lyme disease, as well as ways to treat it.

Staff Credits
Charles Pederson, editor; Adam Lazar, designer; Kim Danger, photo researcher
Cover production by Anne Schafer
Interior production by Stacey Field

Photo Credits
Cover: ©Artville/Don Carstens, left; ©Artville/Clair Alaska, middle; ©Earthstar Stock Inc., right; Stock Market Photo/©Howard Sochurek
Index Stock, 47
International Stock/©Patrick Ramsey, 11; ©Tony Demin, 20
Photo Network/©Bill Terry, 18
Photri, 19, 26/©D&I MacDonald, 41
Unicorn Stock Photos, 54/©Jeff Greenberg, 25, 44; ©Aneal Vohra, 28
Uniphoto/©Bob Daemmrich Photo., Inc 49
Visuals Unlimited/©Ken Greer, 9; ©R. Calentine, 12; ©Jeff J. Daly, 35; ©Robert Clay, 58

A 0 9 8 7 6 5 4 3 2 1

Table of Contents

1	What Is Lyme Disease?	4
2	How People Get Lyme Disease	14
3	Diagnosing Lyme Disease	22
4	Treating Lyme Disease	32
5	Preventing Lyme Disease	42
6	Safety and First Aid	52
	Glossary	60
	For More Information	61
	Useful Addresses and Internet Sites	62
	Index	63

Chapter Overview

For some people, Lyme disease is a minor illness. Other people with Lyme disease may develop serious health problems.

Bacteria cause Lyme disease infection. The bacteria are passed to people through the bite of an infected Lyme tick.

The course of Lyme disease isn't predictable. The symptoms vary from person to person.

There are three stages of Lyme disease: early local disease, disseminated Lyme disease, and chronic or late disease.

Chapter 1

What Is Lyme Disease?

Sydney, Age 14

Sydney liked to take Daisy, the family dog, for walks around the neighborhood. Sometimes they went to a nearby park where Sydney saw wild deer. The deer disappeared when Daisy barked at them.

One day, Sydney developed a swelling in her right knee. It was puffy and tender when touched. Sydney also had a fever and felt tired. Sydney's parents took her to a doctor.

The doctor asked Sydney many questions about her health. Sydney said, "Two weeks ago I banged my right knee during basketball practice. Did that make my knee swell?"

The doctor shook his head. "No. Something else is going on here. I noticed a red rash on the back of your right thigh. I want to run some tests for Lyme disease."

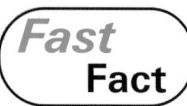

Fast Fact: Lyme disease is the most common tick-carried infection in the United States.

The doctor's information made Sydney and her parents feel hopeful. Lyme disease can be a minor illness. Many people can recover with fast and proper treatment.

Other people can become extremely sick from this disease. They may lose time from school or work. They might not be able to go shopping, play sports, or do other fun things.

Sometimes, Lyme disease results in a physical disability such as arthritis. This causes redness, swelling, stiffness, and pain in a joint in the body. Lyme disease can be chronic, or long-lasting. However, Lyme disease is rarely deadly.

About 12,000 to 15,000 people in the United States get Lyme disease each year. Health experts think these numbers may be much higher. Possibly 10 times as many cases may occur as actually are reported.

Symptoms of Lyme disease can vary from person to person. This may make it hard for doctors to find and report all cases of the disease.

People with Lyme disease can be found throughout the world. The disease affects males and females of any age. Most cases occur in people younger than age 15 and older than 30. Pets such as cats and dogs can get Lyme disease. Like people, they need treatment to be cured.

Ticks and Lyme Disease

Lyme disease is an infection that bacteria cause. The bacterium that causes Lyme disease is named *Borrelia burgdorferi,* or just *Bb*. Bacteria are tiny living things called microorganisms. They are much too small to be seen with the naked eye. Trillions of bacteria are all around us, and most don't cause disease.

Several kinds of ticks can carry *Bb*. All of them are called Lyme ticks in this book. Lyme ticks are tiny creatures that often feed on deer. Sometimes the tiny ticks feed on wild mice and wild birds. *Bb* doesn't harm the ticks or wild animals.

Ticks pass *Bb* to people by biting them. The bacteria enter a person's bloodstream and are carried throughout the body. If the bacteria thrive, Lyme disease can develop. Anyone who lives in or visits an area where Lyme ticks live can become infected.

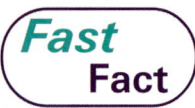

Fast Fact

The central clearing of the EM rash is called a "bull's eye."

Progress Is Unpredictable

Lyme disease can lead to serious illness. It may affect many body parts such as the skin, nervous system, joints, and heart. The course of the disease varies from person to person. This progression can take weeks, months, or even years.

How the disease will progress isn't always easy to predict. Someone may have severe headaches for a week. Then a knee might become swollen. Or the person might feel achy and tired. Another person with Lyme disease may have none of these symptoms.

Stages of Lyme Disease

Lyme disease involves three stages. Each stage is based on the disease's development and symptoms.

Early Local Disease

Lyme disease sometimes begins with a skin rash at the site of a bite from an infected tick. The rash is called *erythema migrans*, or EM. Some people call this a Lyme rash.

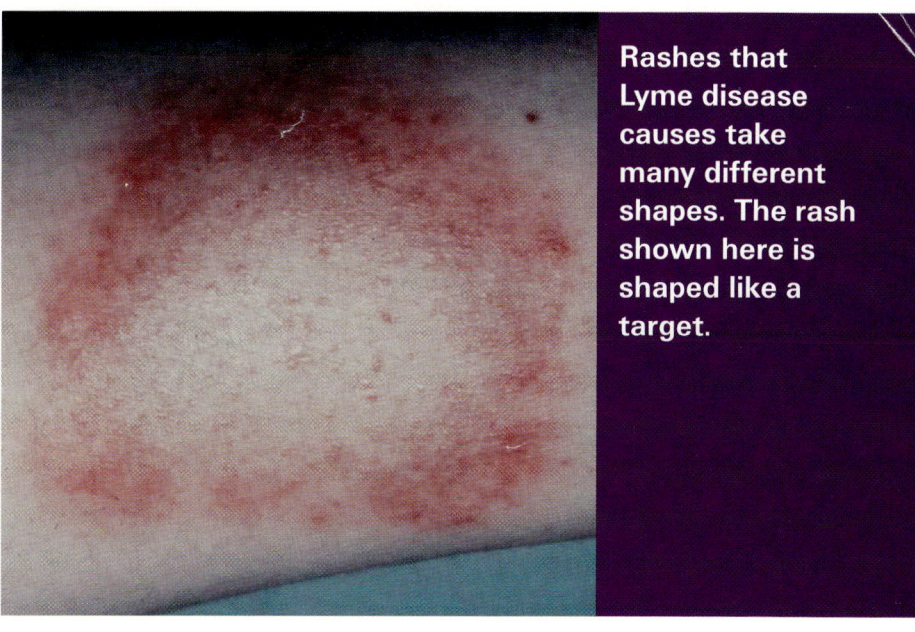

Rashes that Lyme disease causes take many different shapes. The rash shown here is shaped like a target.

An EM rash looks different from other rashes. It may start as a small, red bump that may be raised. The rash expands over a period of days or weeks. It can be as small as the size of a dime. It may grow large enough to cover a person's thigh or back. The center clears as the rash grows. The rash then may form a series of red and paler pink rings. It may look much like a target or sometimes like a bruise if it occurs on darker skin.

The size, shape, and colors of the rash vary. The rash may be large and brightly colored, or it may be small and pale. It may go unnoticed. Some people say it burns, itches, or hurts.

An EM rash can last from one week to several months. It may disappear on its own. However, this doesn't mean the disease is gone. The disease tends to get worse without treatment.

People may have other symptoms along with the rash. They may have headaches, a slight fever, and minor aches and pains. Some people with Lyme disease never develop an EM rash.

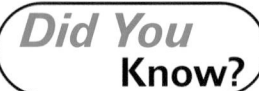

Did You Know? Only since 1994 are doctors required to report all cases of Lyme disease.

Disseminated Lyme Disease

Signs of disseminated Lyme disease appear suddenly. The disease quickly gets worse and spreads to other body parts. Disseminated Lyme disease usually occurs weeks or months after a tick bite.

A person may notice more rashes appearing anywhere on the skin. Some people feel like they have a bad case of the flu. They may have headaches, muscle aches, and a severe fever. Other symptoms include sweating, swollen glands, chills, and sore throat. Many people report feeling tired.

The disease may affect the nervous system at this stage. The bacteria may attack the brain or nerves. The result can be weakness, difficulty walking, or numbness. People sometimes complain of sharp, shooting pains in their arms, legs, or back. The muscles on one or both sides of the face can droop from nerve damage.

The heart may begin to be affected. The heartbeat may become too fast, too slow, or irregular. People may have breathing difficulties or chest pain. Some people feel dizzy.

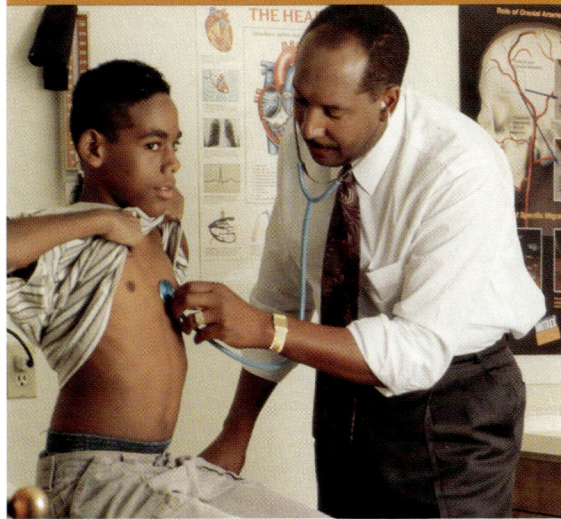

Someone with disseminated Lyme disease may have heart difficulties. A doctor can diagnose this stage of the disease.

Chronic or Late Disease

Chronic Lyme disease affects many body systems. Some people have ongoing rashes and other skin problems. Arthritis is common and may cause one or more joints to become stiff and swollen. The knees often are most affected by Lyme disease. Sometimes the arthritis strikes the shoulders, ankles, and elbows. Muscles also can be damaged, which leads to pain, stiffness, or swelling.

Nerve damage can continue or develop for the first time, which might cause the skin to tingle. Nerve damage also may result in sleeping problems and feeling tired. Some people also report problems with concentration and memory.

Other body systems can be affected. Some people have an upset stomach, throw up, or lose their appetite. Some people report difficulty breathing. They have shortness of breath and need to take quick, shallow gulps of air.

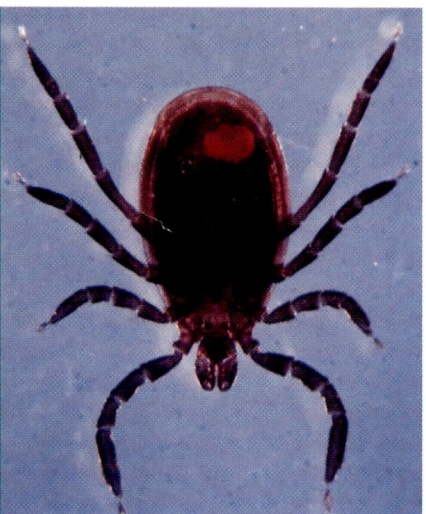

Several ticks may carry Lyme disease. This Lyme tick is called *Ixodes dammini*.

Erik, Age 15

Erik never knew that an infected Lyme tick bit him. He thought he had the flu. His muscle aches and pains never went away. He was tired all the time. He quit the soccer team and stopped taking guitar lessons. The changes in Erik puzzled his family and friends.

Then he told his dad he felt tingling in his feet. He began to have back cramps, and his left ankle swelled. Finally, Erik went to a doctor. Test results showed he had Lyme disease. The doctor thought Erik had gotten the disease many months ago.

A single female tick can lay up to 2,500 eggs at one time.

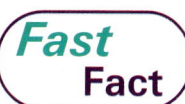

Points to Consider

Some people say untreated Lyme disease is like a time bomb. Do you agree? Why or why not?

Why do you think someone may not see an EM rash?

How do you think you would feel if you found out you had Lyme disease?

Chapter Overview

Lyme disease first was recognized in North America more than 100 years ago. It's been known in Europe for a long time, too.

Infected ticks can transmit the bacteria that cause Lyme disease during three of its four life stages. Some researchers believe the tick must be attached for 24 hours or more before it can transmit bacteria.

Nearly all states and parts of Canada have reported cases of Lyme disease.

Where people live or work can be a risk factor for developing Lyme disease. People in or near woods or areas of tall grass are at risk.

In northern areas, the risk of getting bitten by ticks is highest during warm months. In the South, the risk is constant.

Chapter 2

How People Get Lyme Disease

Byron and Ric, Age 16

It was Saturday afternoon and time to relax. Byron and Ric stretched their legs. They talked about the baseball game they just finished. "What are those little specks on your leg?" Byron pointed to several small black spots on Ric's shin.

Ric took a gulp of soda. "It's just dirt. There was mud in the woods where we looked for the lost ball. I'll wash it off later."

Byron said, "I don't think we should take the chance of getting sick. Let's check for ticks right now."

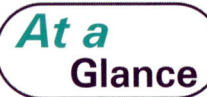

At a Glance

Lyme ticks often feed on deer mice, which also are called white-footed mice. They live in many places such as forests, deserts, mountains, and grassy areas.

In the mid-1970s, something unusual was happening in Lyme, Connecticut, and two nearby towns. A large number of children were diagnosed with a rare type of arthritis. Experts arrived in 1975 to find out why. By May 1976, they counted 39 children and 12 adults with similar symptoms. That summer, experts said these people had a new disease. They called it Lyme disease.

The experts searched the medical history to see if anyone else had written about Lyme disease. They were surprised at what they found. Their "new" disease was actually old. In 1909, a Swedish doctor reported symptoms of Lyme disease in some people. Later, European doctors described people with similar symptoms. The experts learned that Lyme disease has been in the United States for over 100 years.

Health experts studied all this medical history and the people in Lyme. They discovered how the disease is passed. They found a large number of symptoms for Lyme disease. They also found the cause of Lyme disease and how to treat it.

Lyme disease still remains a mystery in some ways. For example, experts don't know how the disease moved from Europe to North America. Exactly why Lyme disease has spread across the United States remains unclear. Also puzzling is why symptoms vary so much from person to person.

Lyme disease may have spread because of reduced use of bug killers on farms and other areas.

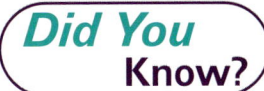

There are probably many reasons why Lyme disease has spread. The number of deer has increased across parts of North America. This increases the number of animals ticks can ride on. Birds and mice can spread the disease from one area to another.

What You Should Know About Ticks

Knowing about ticks helps to understand Lyme disease. Ticks are small arachnids, a group that is related to spiders. Other arachnids include mites and chiggers. All have eight legs, two body parts, and no wings or antennae.

Ticks are parasites. They feed off living animals. In this case, ticks drink the blood of a host. A person, bird, reptile, wild animal, or pet can be a host for ticks.

Ticks feed through their mouthparts, which attach to a host's skin. Tiny hooks or barbs cover the mouthparts. These keep the tick firmly attached while it feeds. If infected with *Bb*, a tick can transmit these bacteria to its host.

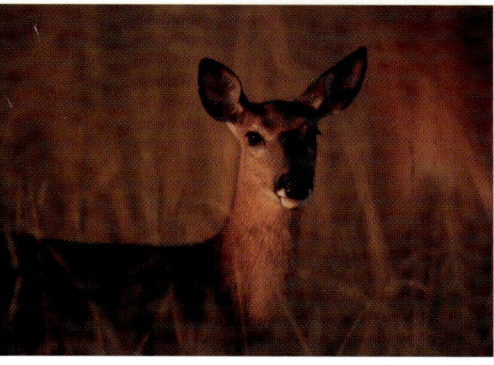

Deer, mice, and birds are common hosts for Lyme ticks.

Scientists don't fully understand how ticks find a host. Ticks have no eyes or ears. They must rely on other senses to know when a person or animal is nearby. Young and mature ticks wait on grass, shrubs, and bushes. When people or animals brush by, ticks crawl or drop onto the skin. Claws and sticky pads on their feet help ticks latch onto the skin.

Ticks go through four life stages: egg, larva, nymph, and adult. A tick can spread infection during the larva, nymph, and adult stages. Ticks at these life stages feed on hosts. An average tick lives about two years.

Lyme Ticks

More than 850 different kinds of ticks exist in the world. About 100 of these can transmit microorganisms like bacteria to people. The most common carrier of Lyme disease in the United States is the deer tick. Other carriers are the black-legged tick, the bear tick, and western black-legged tick. The number of ticks carrying Lyme disease varies by location. It may range from none to 90 percent of the ticks.

Tick larvae are about the size of the period at the end of this sentence. Nymphs are a bit larger than larvae. Adult Lyme ticks are flat and about the size of a sesame seed until they have fed. Males are black, and females are reddish with a black spot that looks like a shield near the head. Lyme ticks may grow to about the size and color of a raisin after they have fed.

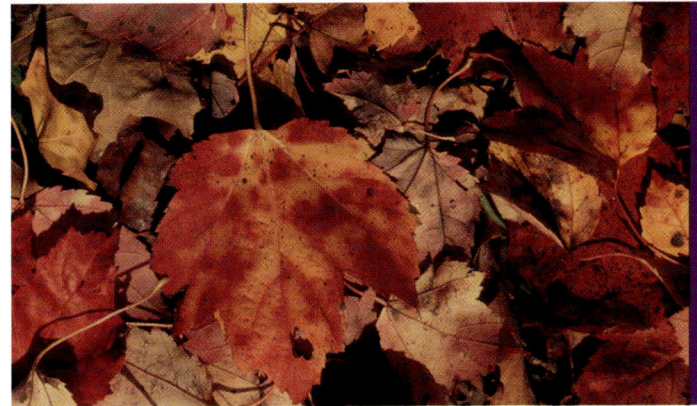

When larvae finish feeding, they drop off their host and may hide under fallen leaves. The larvae rest as they mature into nymphs.

How Lyme Disease Is Transmitted

Bacteria carried in the digestive tubes of ticks cause Lyme disease. Tick eggs hatch into larvae in spring. The larvae may get *Bb* by feeding on the blood of infected mice and deer. Larvae drop to the ground after they have eaten and hide under fallen and dead leaves.

The larvae mature into nymphs the next spring. Nymphs look like tiny adult ticks but aren't fully mature. They are most active in late May, June, and July. As during the other stages of Lyme ticks, nymphs feed on blood. If they carry *Bb*, they can infect people. After their meal, nymphs rest and mature into adults over the winter.

Adult ticks feed mostly on deer, mice, and sometimes birds. However, they may feed on other animals, including humans. Ticks transmit bacteria only when they feed. Males may attach to people, but sometimes they don't feed. Female ticks are more likely to transmit Lyme disease. They must feed on blood to produce eggs.

After ticks feed, they usually drop into the leaves on the ground. Male ticks die after they mate with females. Female ticks live through the winter, lay eggs in the spring, and die. The cycle continues when the eggs hatch.

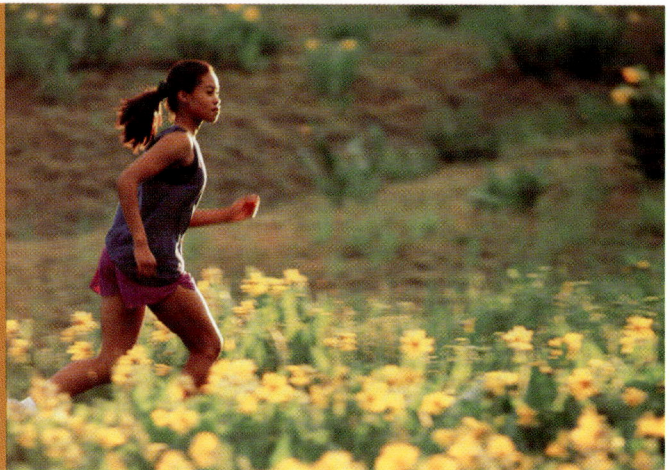

Exercising in grassy areas may be a high-risk activity. Tall grass may be home to Lyme ticks.

Even if a tick carries *Bb*, it may not transfer bacteria. Experiments show that the tick must attach for at least 24 hours before it can transmit bacteria. People have more chance of getting Lyme disease if the tick gets a full feeding. Nymphs feed from one to three days. Adults feed up to a week.

People at High Risk

Some people may be at a higher risk than others to contract Lyme disease. People's home or workplace is a risk factor. Lyme disease is reported in 49 states of the United States and many parts of Canada.

People who go to places in or near wooded areas are at high risk of tick bites. However, both city and rural areas can be risk areas. This is particularly true if mice, deer, or other Lyme tick hosts visit the area. Places with tall grass also may be homes for ticks. The side of roads or the grassy areas around beaches may contain ticks.

People can develop Lyme disease any time of the year. In areas with cold winters, the risk is much higher during warm months. That's because people are outside more when the weather is warm. At the same time, nymphs and ticks are more active in warm weather. In some southern areas, ticks can pass Lyme disease at any time.

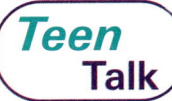

"My parents read about Lyme disease. They were scared to go to our neighbor's house. It's on a nice, clear lake with plenty of beach. I told them Lyme ticks usually wait on long grass, trees, or leaves. They don't live in sand. So don't worry, and let's start packing!"—Tony, age 15

"I was surprised when I tested positive for Lyme disease. No one I knew had it. It wasn't discussed in my health class, and I didn't know anything about it. My doctor said that a Lyme tick bit me, though I don't remember seeing a tick.

"I live in a suburb and never see deer. The doctor said ticks can live in grassy areas near woods. I'm not sure how I got Lyme disease. A month ago, I spent a couple hours looking along a road for cans to recycle in the area. Lots of tall grass grew there. That's probably how ticks found me."

Iris, Age 16

Points to Consider

How do you think you could find out if your area has many Lyme ticks?

Do you think the risk of getting Lyme disease is higher in Michigan or Florida? Explain.

Why would an outdoor worker be more at risk than an indoor worker to get Lyme disease?

Chapter Overview

Early diagnosis of Lyme disease is important. The sooner treatment begins, the better the chance that a person with the disease will recover.

Common symptoms of early local Lyme disease include an enlarging rash, fever, headache, pain in joints and bones, chills, and stiff neck. Typical symptoms of chronic Lyme disease include arthritis and muscle weakness. Lyme disease also can cause loss of control of face muscles and irregular heartbeat.

Diagnosing Lyme disease begins with gathering a description of symptoms, the person's medical history, and a general examination. Blood tests can reveal the presence of Lyme disease. A test of the fluid in an affected joint can help confirm the diagnosis.

Chapter 3

Diagnosing Lyme Disease

Han, Age 16

Han was on the school's soccer and baseball teams. He ran three miles a day and lifted weights. He earned top scores on his tests and hoped to graduate with honors. That spring, Han decided to change where he ran. He mapped out a new course through a nearby forested area each day. It was a nice change. One day, he found three red, round rashes on his leg. He went to the doctor, who gave Han a lotion to put on the rashes.

Han went back to the doctor a month later. The rashes were still there. He also had a stiff neck and lots of headaches. He felt tired all the time and had stopped running. His grades were slipping. "It's some flu bug you picked up. You just need a few weeks of rest to feel better," said the doctor.

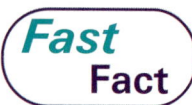

Fast Fact: Lyme disease is one of the fastest-growing infectious diseases in North America.

This doctor was unfamiliar with Lyme disease and made the wrong diagnosis, or determination, of Han's disease. Early diagnosis of Lyme disease is important. People in any stage of Lyme disease need treatment right away. Without treatment, their symptoms often get worse.

Symptoms of Lyme Disease

A diagnosis of Lyme disease usually comes about in one of two ways. People with early local Lyme disease may feel sick. They may notice something unusual about their body. They go to the doctor to find out the cause of their symptoms. Sometimes the person has no early symptoms of Lyme disease.

People with disseminated or chronic Lyme disease often have several symptoms, usually involving their skin. Arthritis and nerve or heart problems are common, too. Doctors discover the Lyme disease during an examination and through medical tests.

A visit to the doctor is needed if you suspect you have Lyme disease. A doctor can discover the disease through medical testing.

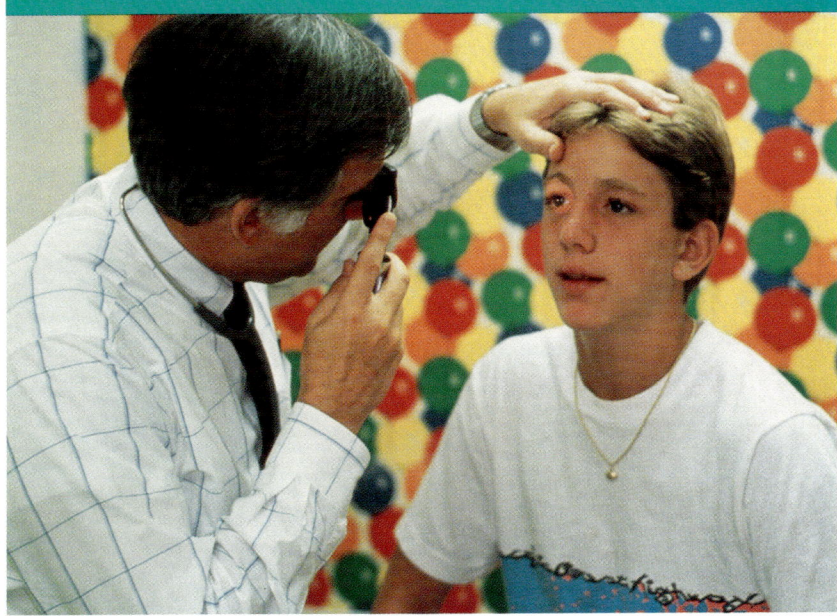

Han showed symptoms of early local Lyme disease. Common early symptoms include the following:

Enlarging rash. The rash may have a ring of lighter and darker colors. The rash may look like a red target, or it may take many other shapes and colors.

Headache

Chills

Neck stiffness

Fever

Muscle aches and pains

Joint pain

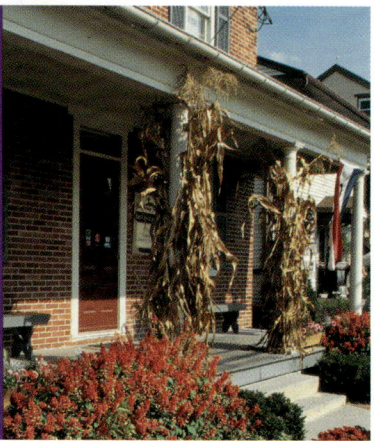

Woods and forests aren't the only places where Lyme ticks may live. Even areas within cities can harbor them.

If left untreated, Han may develop more serious symptoms. Disseminated and chronic symptoms of Lyme disease include the following:

- Arthritis, especially in one or both knees
- Weakness
- Changes in feeling in any part of the skin
- Loss of control of face muscles
- Irregular heartbeat
- Memory loss
- Difficulty concentrating
- Changes in mood or sleep habits

Difficulties in Diagnosis

Lyme disease isn't always easy to recognize. It's sometimes called the "great imitator" because its many symptoms can seem like those of other illnesses. Like Han's doctor, medical professionals unfamiliar with Lyme disease may miss a correct diagnosis. Some people need to visit a doctor more than once before their disease is correctly diagnosed. A correct diagnosis may take weeks, months, or even years.

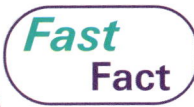

Most children who develop Lyme disease have one or more EM rashes.

For example, Han's doctor decided Han simply had a rash. Later, the doctor thought Han might have had a bad case of the flu.

Diagnosing Lyme disease can be difficult for another reason. One person can go from a rash to severe arthritis within months. Another person can go from no rash to serious heart problems in just weeks. The disease is different for each individual.

Gathering Physical Information

Diagnosing Lyme disease involves several steps. The diagnosis is based on the person's physical signs and symptoms and medical tests. Lyme disease also may be diagnosed if a person has been in an area where Lyme ticks might live.

Doctors first ask about a person's physical symptoms. They also take the person's medical history. They want to know about the person's health in the past. They ask about the person's travel history. People in non-Lyme disease areas may have traveled to woods or grassy areas filled with ticks. Sometimes people can bring the doctor the tick that bit them. All this information helps to explain the person's symptoms.

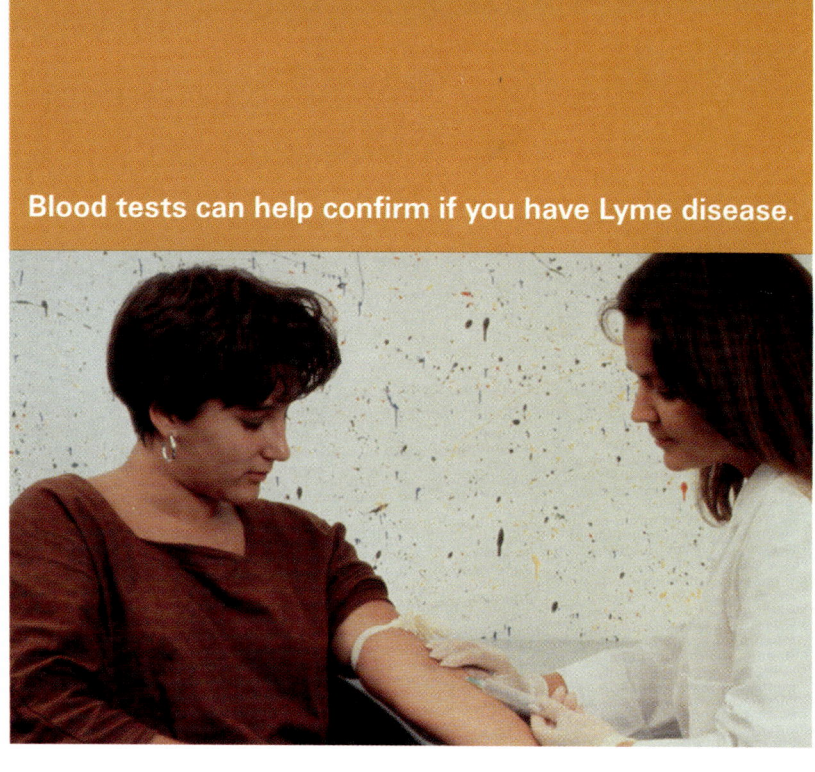

Blood tests can help confirm if you have Lyme disease.

The next step is a physical exam. Doctors observe the person's general health. They check blood pressure, temperature, and heart rate. They look over the skin for any rashes.

Medical Tests

Blood tests can help in diagnosing Lyme disease. A number of different blood tests can identify the bacteria.

The immune system protects the body from disease. It creates antibodies to fight specific bacteria, including Lyme disease. Antibodies are special cells that fight infection. Laboratory technicians, a nurse, or doctor takes some blood and looks at it under a microscope. They can tell if the Lyme disease bacteria antibodies are present.

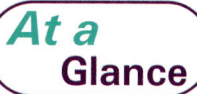

Bacteria come in three shapes. Some are round balls, some are twisted spirals, and others are straight rods. The bacteria that cause Lyme disease are spiral-shaped. They are called spirochetes.

Understanding the results of a Lyme disease antibody test can be tricky at times. Different doctors may interpret the blood test results differently. Sometimes a blood test isn't accurate for Lyme disease. Doctors may require more than one type of blood test to get correct information. The blood tests may not detect early local Lyme disease. The person may have to get another blood test a month or so later.

To further aid in diagnosing, doctors may remove some fluid from a person's swollen or painful joint. They then examine this fluid. The results of this exam can confirm the diagnosis of Lyme disease.

Doctors may do a spinal tap, or lumbar puncture, to determine if Lyme disease is affecting the nervous system. For this test, a doctor withdraws a small amount of spinal fluid from the spinal cord. The fluid can show if the disease has spread to the brain and nervous system. Spinal taps also may be done to check the progress of treatment. They can be painful.

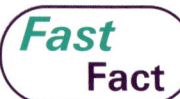

Fast Fact

Over 155,000 cases of Lyme disease have been reported in the United States since 1982.

Mistakes Can Happen

Each of the following teens had Lyme disease but was told he or she had something else:

Peter, age 14, was diagnosed with arthritis when his knees and right ankle swelled. He told the doctor he had other symptoms. He had a lot of headaches and a stiff neck. The doctor insisted the only thing wrong was arthritis.

Sameer, age 19, was shocked when he was told he had multiple sclerosis. With this disease, the nervous system degenerates. People can lose the ability to walk as they lose control of muscles. Sameer did not respond to a year of treatment for multiple sclerosis. He wondered if he needed to see a different doctor to get another diagnosis.

Hannah, age 17, no longer could drive. The once-active teen had tremors, or body shakes. She felt dizzy much of the time. She also had difficulty learning, and her grades dropped. The doctor asked Hannah if she was using drugs. Drug abuse could be causing the problems. Hannah said no. In fact, Hannah had been involved in an antidrug program at school. Hannah's symptoms puzzled the doctor.

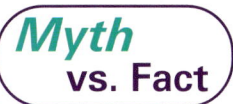

Myth: Lyme disease is contagious. You can get Lyme disease from someone who is infected with the disease.

Fact: Lyme disease isn't contagious. You can't get Lyme disease from another person or an infected animal. No one has developed Lyme disease from the air, food, or water. Lyme disease isn't spread through sexual contact.

If you think you might have Lyme disease, tell your doctor. You might have your parents ask your doctor for a Lyme disease test. You even could show your doctor this book.

Points to Consider

Why might it be easy to misdiagnose Lyme disease?

Which Lyme disease test do you think would be the hardest to take? How could you prepare for it?

How do you think you would react if you found out you had Lyme disease?

Chapter Overview

Treatment for Lyme disease aims to kill the bacteria so they never return. Doctors consider people recovered if they are totally free of symptoms.

Most people treated for Lyme disease return to a healthy life. A small number of people develop ongoing symptoms. This condition is called post-Lyme disease syndrome.

Antibiotic drugs are the main treatment for Lyme disease. Treatment plans vary from person to person depending on symptoms and how the person reacts to the drugs.

Treatment for Lyme disease may cause unpleasant side effects. These include diarrhea, constipation, stomach upset, stomach cramps, loss of appetite, headache, and sensitivity to sunlight.

People with chronic Lyme disease experience high levels of stress. Their family does, too. The support of others is helpful.

Chapter 4

Treating Lyme Disease

Treatment for Lyme disease aims at complete recovery. Doctors consider people recovered when they are totally free of Lyme disease symptoms. Treatment isn't always simple because each person is different. Some people with the bacteria never develop the disease. Or they have a mild, brief illness that disappears without treatment. Many other people need treatment to recover.

When symptoms disappear and then return later, it's called a relapse. The bacteria remain in the body months or even years after the infection and treatment. Doctors aren't sure how the bacteria can hide so well. This kind of infection is difficult to treat because it's hard to kill the bacteria.

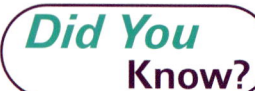

Did You Know? Antibiotics work in two ways. Some kill bacteria directly. Other antibiotics interfere with the bacteria's ability to reproduce and grow. This gives the immune system time to kill the bacteria.

It's important to begin treatment of Lyme disease as soon as possible. Early treatment provides the best chance of complete recovery and helps prevent damage to the body.

No standard treatment plan exists for Lyme disease. Doctors design a treatment plan to fit each person's needs. They consider the person's age, symptoms, and general health. They also consider how many and which body systems are affected.

Success of Treatment

Most people treated for Lyme disease return to a healthy life. Few people die from Lyme disease.

Even with treatment, a small percentage of people develop symptoms that don't go away. They may have constant pain, memory problems, and a tired feeling. This condition is called post-Lyme disease syndrome, or PLDS. Bacteria that remain after treatment may cause PLDS. Sometimes the infection can cause the immune system to work incorrectly. This improper functioning also may cause PLDS.

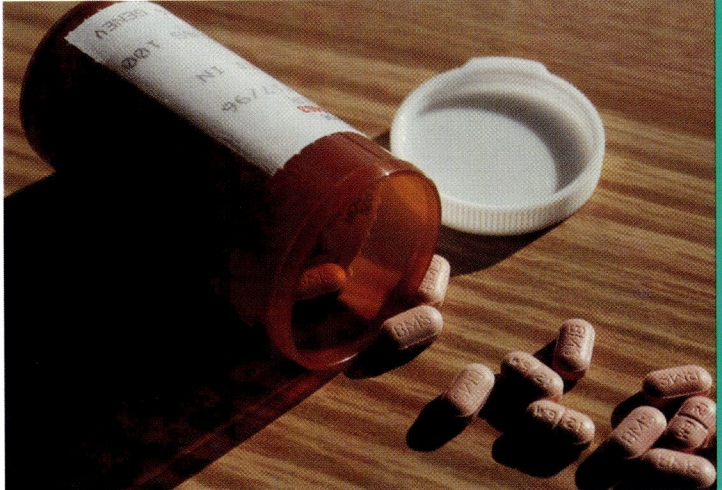

Antibiotics fight Lyme disease. This medicine usually comes in the form of prescription pills.

Antibiotics

Antibiotics are the usual form of treatment for Lyme disease. These powerful drugs work to kill unwanted bacteria. Antibiotics don't attack healthy body cells.

Four types of antibiotics fight Lyme disease. The doctor determines which type is best, based on the person's age, symptoms, and other factors. Some antibiotics can be used by teens age 12 and up only. Some are best for early Lyme disease. Others are used for people with late or chronic Lyme disease.

People receive different doses, or amounts, of antibiotics. The doses are often greater than for bacterial infections such as strep throat. People usually take the antibiotics by mouth in pill form. Sometimes the drug is put into the muscles or blood vessels with a needle.

Stages of Treatment

Doctors usually begin treating Lyme disease with antibiotics for two to four weeks. The length of a treatment plan depends on the disease stage and symptoms.

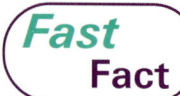

Children under the age of 12 can't use some antibiotics. These drugs can cause stained or poorly formed teeth.

Early Lyme disease can require two or three weeks of treatment. The person usually takes the antibiotics as a pill. This can be done at home or most other places.

Acute or chronic Lyme disease is more difficult to treat. At this point, the disease has been carried throughout the person's body. The bacteria are in many body cells. Doctors may combine two or three antibiotics for tougher cases of Lyme disease. These antibiotics are taken at the same time.

Sometimes a person must take antibiotics for months or even years. In these cases, the person may get shots of the drugs. The person gets the shots in the doctor's office, in a clinic, or at home. Sometimes the disease affects the brain, nerves, or heart. Then the person would go into the hospital and be treated with antibiotics dripped directly into a blood vessel.

Most people with Lyme disease begin to improve soon after starting antibiotics. It usually takes two to six weeks of treatment to see major improvement.

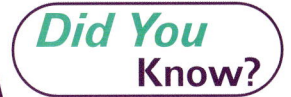

The U.S. government estimates that thousands of Lyme disease cases aren't diagnosed, treated, or even reported. This is often because the disease easily can be mistaken for many other illnesses.

Laurel, Age 14

Laurel had chronic Lyme disease. The doctor explained that the treatment plan would be in stages. Laurel first got antibiotic shots for four weeks. Her mother gave Laurel the shots at home. Laurel got used to the shots after a few days. The needle pain lasted only a short time.

Laurel's symptoms didn't improve. The doctor prescribed another two weeks of antibiotics. Laurel still had most of her symptoms. Finally, the doctor had Laurel take antibiotics in pill form. She took them for a few months before the doctor said she was recovered.

Side Effects of Antibiotics

Antibiotics can cause unpleasant side effects, or unwanted results. Each antibiotic tends to produce its own side effects. Common side effects include diarrhea, stomach upset and cramps, loss of appetite, and headache. Some people get a metallic taste in their mouth.

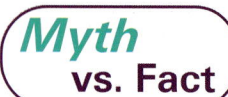

Myth: Heavy or long-term use of antibiotics can destroy a person's immune system.

Fact: Using antibiotics for even a long time won't destroy the body's immune system. A person isn't left defenseless against other infections.

Antibiotics can trigger vaginitis by disturbing the natural balance of bacteria in female genitals. These are the sex organs. Vaginitis causes the female genitals to itch, burn, and turn red. Sometimes a bad-smelling fluid may come from the genitals.

If a female is using pills to prevent pregnancy, she also should use another form of birth control. Antibiotics reduce the effectiveness of the pills.

People on antibiotic treatment for more than two weeks need to watch what they eat. The drugs can affect the balance of bacteria in the large intestine, where many harmless bacteria live. Antibiotics can change the consistency of undigested food to diarrhea. This is a semisolid waste that's passed from the body. Doctors can advise a person on which foods to eat or avoid.

Some people who take antibiotics may find their symptoms getting worse. This is a sign that the drug is attacking the Lyme disease bacteria. The bacteria react to the drug, and the immune system overreacts to the bacteria. This reaction can last from two days to two weeks before the person begins to feel better.

> **Fast Fact**
>
> Lyme disease occurs more often in children than in adults.

Sometimes people are allergic to an antibiotic. The body rejects and reacts to the drug in the body. An allergic reaction may include skin problems such as a rash or hives. People may have breathing problems, vomiting, fever, or sore throat. Numbness, tingling, or burning in arms, hands, legs, or feet might occur.

People with Lyme disease arthritis need drugs to reduce the swelling and pain of affected joints. Other drugs treat heart and nervous system problems.

Finding Support

People with chronic Lyme disease or people who don't respond well to therapy may experience high levels of stress. Their family often feels stressed, too. Taking care of a seriously ill family member can be exhausting. It's difficult to keep up with jobs and other responsibilities. There are many things to worry about. Fortunately, hundreds of support groups exist across North America. They support people with Lyme disease. Their family also can receive support.

Several organizations also can help. These organizations support research on Lyme disease and provide free information about the disease and treatment methods. They can find local support groups for people with Lyme disease. They give referrals to doctors who specialize in Lyme disease. For information about these organizations, see the section Useful Addresses and Internet Sites on page 62.

The Centers for Disease Control and Prevention (CDC) collects Lyme disease information for the U.S. government. The CDC also provides information about the disease and treatment methods. Many state public health departments and some cities provide information about Lyme disease.

Different organizations can give you information about Lyme disease. You can call many of them for free.

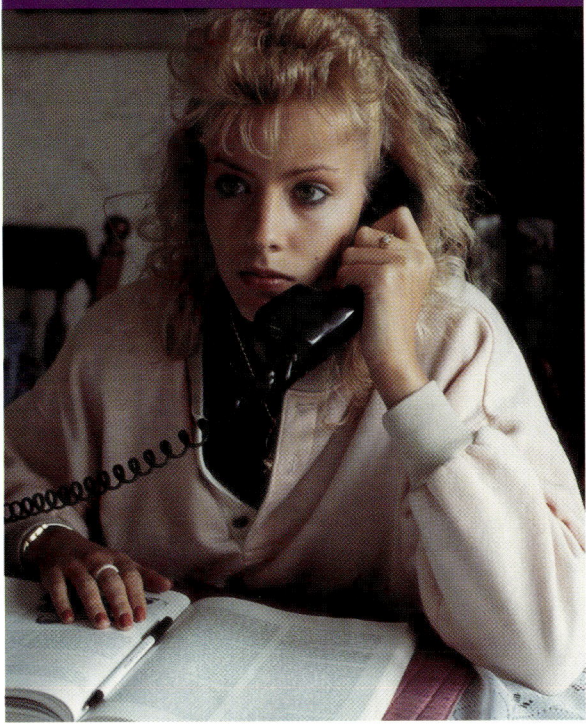

Points to Consider

What do you think the worst thing would be about being treated for Lyme disease? Why?

Some schools don't allow students to carry prescription drugs. Why do you think that's true?

Does your school allow students to carry prescription drugs? If you don't know your school's policy, how could you find out?

How could you help someone with chronic Lyme disease during his or her treatment?

Chapter Overview

The best way to avoid Lyme disease is to stay away from ticks. Avoid areas where ticks are likely to live. This is most important during warm months.

Wearing the right kinds of clothing can help keep ticks away from the skin. It's best to wear shoes, long pants, long-sleeved tops, and a hat or scarf. People can spray clothing with a tick repellent. This helps to keep ticks from attaching.

Lyme disease vaccine can help prevent Lyme disease. The vaccine isn't recommended for everyone and doesn't prevent all cases of Lyme disease.

Chapter 5

Preventing Lyme Disease

Terry and John, Age 17

Terry and John had taken a fun, long, and hot hike. Now the two friends studied a map. John took it and sat on the ground. "Look! Here's a shortcut home. Let's take that. We can save time and not walk so far."

Terry shook his head. "There are a lot of trees that way that could be filled with ticks. Let's just stay on the main path. It's wider and will be easier to stay in the center. And John, get off the ground! Look at those leaves you're sitting in. You're probably crawling with ticks."

It's not always easy to avoid ticks. Even being in your own garden could expose you to Lyme disease.

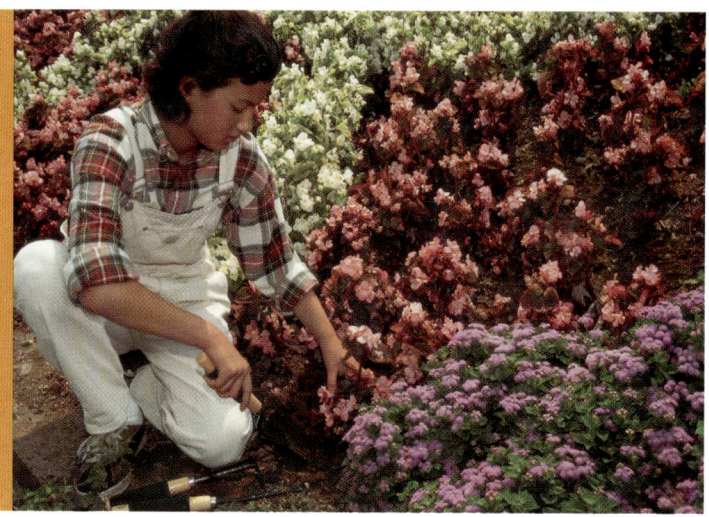

The best way to avoid getting Lyme disease is to stay away from ticks. This can be difficult. Ticks are spreading across North America, and so is the disease. Ticks live in the woods, brush, bushes, and high grasses. They are common where wooded areas and nearby grasslands come together. They also can be found in the yards of city homes.

Even being inside is not always complete protection. A tick can ride on a person's clothing, crawl out, and bite someone. Or a tick can hide in the fur of a pet and latch onto someone nearby.

Being Prepared

The best way to avoid tick bites is to be prepared. People can do many things to keep ticks away.

Avoid Tick Areas

If possible, avoid going into areas likely to harbor ticks. This is most important during warm months when ticks like to feed. Ticks favor moist, shady areas. They prefer leaf litter and low-growing bushes, shrubs, and trees. They also prefer high grasses. Usually, deer or mice must live in the area to act as hosts for Lyme ticks.

State and local health departments can supply information on areas where ticks are common. Contact state and local park workers and county extension services.

Dress Properly and Keep Clean
The right kinds of clothing can help keep ticks away from the skin. Ticks move up from the ground, shrubs, or grass. It's important to wear shoes that cover the feet completely. Shoes, sneakers, or boots work best. Wearing sandals isn't a good idea.

Outdoors, wear long pants and a top with long sleeves. Tuck the top into the pants. Tight cuffs and collars are best for shirts and pants. Also tuck the bottoms of pant legs into socks or boots or put a rubber band around cuffs.

Wearing a hat or scarf keeps ticks off the hair and scalp. Light-colored clothing makes it easier to see dark ticks. Tightly woven fabrics help, too. Ticks have a harder time attaching onto smooth fabric.

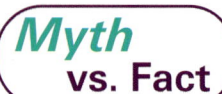

Myth: Ticks move around by flying, jumping, or hopping.

Fact: Ticks don't fly, jump, or hop. They crawl up things or animals, usually 3 feet (.9 meters) or less from the ground.

After returning from a tick area, be sure to check your entire body for ticks. Take a shower if you can. The running water can wash off unattached ticks.

Wash and dry clothing worn outdoors. Ticks can hide in clothing, especially pockets and folds. Wear freshly cleaned clothing whenever you go out.

Use Tick Repellent

Spray clothing with a tick repellent, which keeps ticks away. Tick repellents that work best contain a substance called deet. Tick repellents with deet help prevent ticks from attaching.

However, certain risks are associated with using deet. Never spray repellants with deet directly on the skin, especially the face. Deet can burn the eyes or lips. Young children shouldn't use tick repellents that contain deet. Deet repellents may cause side effects such as itching, a rash, or hives. If this happens, wash the affected area and clothing immediately after returning indoors. Other tick repellents without deet are available. These repellents don't have the same risks as deet.

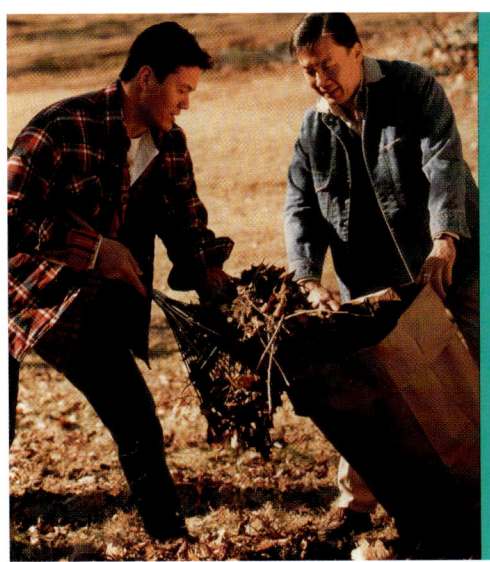

Keep your property free of dead leaves or other litter. This can reduce areas that Lyme ticks and their hosts like.

Experts recommend spraying socks, pants, top, and hat or bandanna that can be worn around the head. Be careful because deet may damage some plastics and other artificial fabrics. Wash the repellent off yourself after being outside.

Keep Property Free of Ticks
Experts advise keeping wildlife away from homes and yards. Don't put food out for animals to eat. Having bird feeders or birdbaths can be risky. Birds can carry ticks. Other animals such as mice, which carry Lyme ticks, can eat the food or drink the water. They may bring their ticks with them.

There are other ways to reduce the number of ticks at home. If possible, remove rock walls. Don't sit on them. Ticks can be found in rock walls.

Keep grass cut short and shrubs and bushes trimmed. Remove leaf litter. Get rid of brush or woodpiles near the house. These actions help reduce areas that deer, mice, and ticks like. More sunlight can enter, which keeps the area dry and warm. Ticks prefer shady, moist areas.

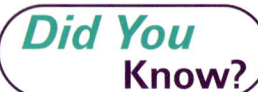

Did You Know? Lyme ticks may be active during winter months. This may be true even in places with cold winters.

Various stores sell products that help keep an area free of ticks. Some products are sprayed on shrubs and bushes or in picnic areas. Other products are sprinkled around the base of shrubs. Another product comes in tubes stuffed with cotton balls that are treated with a chemical substance. The tubes are placed under bushes. Mice use the cotton balls to make nests. The chemical substance kills ticks when they fall into it, yet the mice remain unharmed.

Read product labels before using any substances for ticks. The label explains how to use the product, what it does, and how long it lasts.

Lyme Disease Vaccine

Lyme disease vaccine can help prevent Lyme disease. This liquid contains parts of Lyme bacteria. The vaccine causes the body to produce antibodies against Lyme disease. The vaccine can't cause infection to develop because it has no complete bacteria.

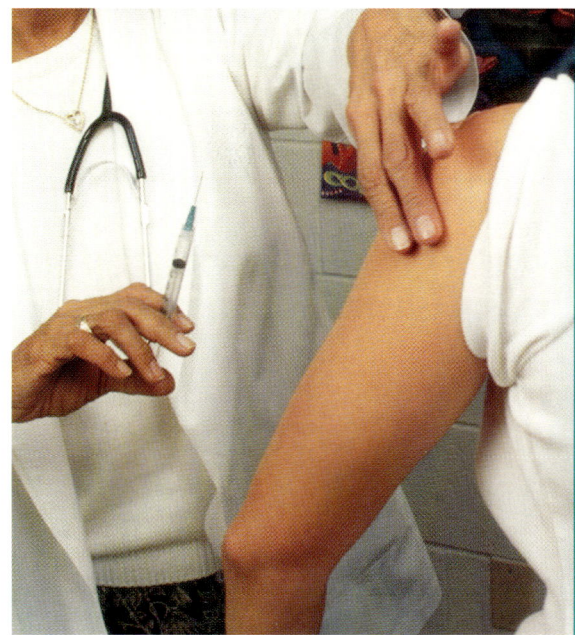

The vaccine against Lyme disease is injected with a needle. A person needs three shots for best protection.

The Lyme disease vaccine is injected by needle. It's given in three doses over the course of one year. The first dose is usually given in January, February, or March. The second dose follows 1 month later. The third dose is given 12 months after the first.

People who live in or travel to areas where Lyme disease is a problem may want the vaccine. Other vaccine candidates are people who spend time in wooded, brushy, or overgrown areas. People who hike, camp, or visit cabins may want to get the vaccine. Even if someone has had Lyme disease before, he or she still can get it again.

Only people between the ages of 15 and 70 can get the vaccine. Children under 15 and pregnant women shouldn't get the vaccine. People with some types of arthritis or heart problems aren't candidates for the vaccine. Doctors don't recommend the vaccine if people are at low or no risk for Lyme disease. These people don't live, work, or play in areas with Lyme ticks.

Problems With the Lyme Disease Vaccine

Any vaccine can cause mild to serious problems. However, the risk of a vaccine causing serious harm or death is small. Most people who have gotten the Lyme disease vaccine have had no problems.

Some mild problems can occur. You may feel sore where the shot was given. The area can turn red or swell a little. Or you may feel mild flu-like symptoms. You may have muscle aches, joint pains, fever, and chills.

The vaccine isn't 100 percent effective. It provides up to 78 percent protection against Lyme disease. You may still get Lyme disease even after receiving all the injections. Experts don't yet know how long protection lasts. The Lyme disease vaccine doesn't protect against other diseases passed by ticks.

Into the Future

Lizards may protect some areas from Lyme disease. The Western fence lizard has a blood protein that kills Lyme bacteria as the tick feeds. The protein doesn't harm the tick or lizard. Lizards can't survive in colder areas, so scientists are looking for other animals to help control Lyme disease.

Points to Consider

Why do you think Lyme disease occurs more often in children than in adults?

After reading this chapter, will you dress differently in wooded or grassy areas? How?

Do you know anyone who has gotten the Lyme disease vaccine? If so, did the person react to the vaccine?

Why do you think the Lyme vaccine isn't recommended for people under age 15?

Chapter Overview

Always check for ticks after returning from a tick area. Ticks' favorite hiding places are the hair, scalp, neck, and ears. They also like to hide between the legs and behind the knees.

Remove an attached tick right away. Use tweezers with a fine point. You may want to have an attached tick tested for the Lyme disease bacteria.

Pets can get Lyme disease from ticks. Pets also can bring ticks in from outside and put people at risk for infection. Pet owners need to check their pets for ticks regularly.

Chapter 6

Safety and First Aid

Jarell and Manuela, Ages 15 and 16

Jarell finished weeding her area in the flower garden. She walked over to help Manuela.

"Thanks," said Manuela. She rolled up her shirtsleeves. "Look, there's a walking freckle on my right arm. What is it?"

"Isn't that just a speck of dirt?" said Jarrell. She moved closer. "Oh, you're right, it's moving. It could be a tick."

Even after taking precautions, ticks still can crawl onto someone and bite the skin. Pets also can be at risk for getting Lyme disease. First aid, or immediate care, can help a person or pet avoid developing Lyme disease.

Boots with pants tucked into the top help protect against ticks. However, you still should check your entire body after spending time in tick areas.

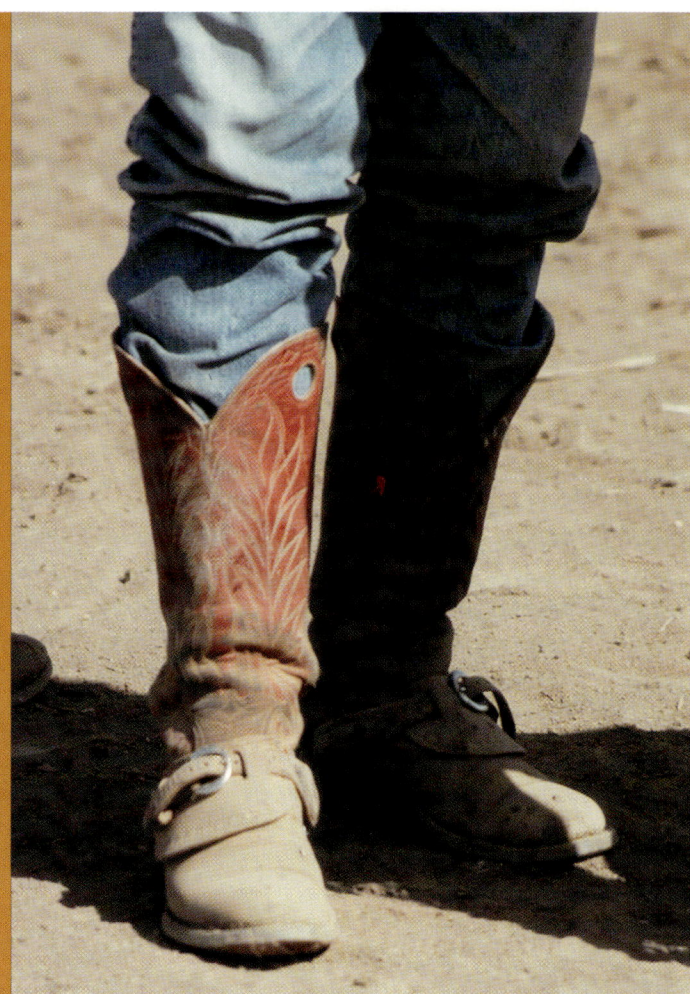

Finding Ticks

Ticks are small and often hard to notice. They may look like dirt. Many people never realize they have been bitten because tick bites are often painless.

For these reasons, always check your entire body after being in tick areas. Taking a shower is a good idea, too, as the running water may wash off unattached ticks.

> **Did You Know?**
> Pharmacies and medical supply stores sell tweezers to remove ticks.

An attached tick often feels like a small scab. Ticks often hide in the hair and scalp, on the neck, and in and behind the ears. Using a comb with fine teeth will help find adult ticks in the scalp and hair. Ticks also crawl into the underarms, between the legs, behind the knees, and onto the lower legs and arms. Use a mirror to check your back, or have someone else look.

Ticks often crawl around before they attach to the skin. Ticks may look like a moving freckle or a sesame seed. They may be as large as a raisin. Nymphs are the hardest to spot because they are the smallest form of the tick.

Remove any tick right away. If you can, wear rubber or latex gloves, or place a tissue or leaf between the fingers. Then pick up the tick. Don't prick, crush, or burn it. The tick might release infected fluids. Put the tick into a plastic bag or other container, seal it, and throw it away. Wash your hands after handling a tick.

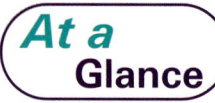

At a Glance

There are wrong ways to remove an attached tick. Don't get ticks out of the skin by burning or coating them with anything. Using nail polish remover, petroleum jelly, or butter isn't a good idea. These methods don't work.

Skye and Joe, Ages 13 and 15

Skye had a tick attached to her back. Joe finished putting on a pair of rubber gloves and moved behind Skye.

"Remember what we talked about, Joe?" Skye said. "Don't twist or yank the tick out. If you do, the mouthparts could stay in my back. Or the tick could release some infected fluids."

Joe stood in front of his sister. He held the tick in the tweezers. "While you were talking, you had a successful operation!"

Removing an Attached Tick

It's important to remove an attached tick properly and as soon as possible. It usually takes just a few seconds. Use tweezers with a fine rounded point. Don't use eyebrow tweezers. They can squeeze the tick and cause infected fluids to enter the skin.

Use the tweezers to grasp the mouthparts of the tick near your skin. This is where the tick is attached. Pull the tick out in a steady, gentle motion. Put the tick into a plastic bag or other container with a lid and seal it.

Always wash hands with hot water and soap. Clean the bite area with rubbing alcohol. Then wash the tweezers with soap and hot water.

Sometimes the mouthparts of the tick break off in the skin. Use a clean needle to remove this part right away. Call a doctor right away if a tick or its mouthparts can't be removed.

Consider getting ticks tested for the Lyme disease bacteria. It's best to keep ticks alive for the testing lab. Ticks need moisture. To keep a tick alive, add two small blades of grass to the container. Or wet a small piece of tissue with water and put it into the container. Seal the container and refrigerate until testing time.

A variety of places offer tick testing. State and local health departments or a university can suggest testing places. A veterinarian, or animal doctor, also can test ticks for Lyme disease bacteria.

When to Call a Doctor

If a tick bites you, take precautions in case Lyme disease develops. Write down where the tick attached and the general state of your health. Keep this information on a calendar or in a notebook. Watch for changes in your health for a month. Write down anything unusual and call a doctor if symptoms occur.

It's usually not necessary to call a doctor after a tick bite. Most likely, you won't get sick. If symptoms develop, see a doctor right away and bring the tick. The doctor will send it to a lab to be examined.

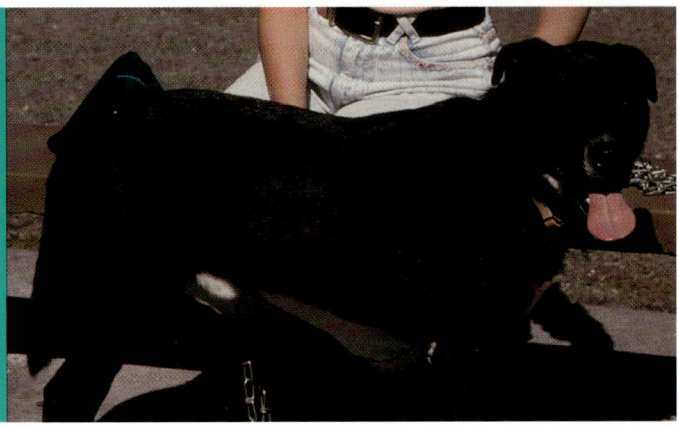

Pets may carry Lyme ticks indoors. Pets themselves also may develop Lyme disease. Antibiotics will help them to fight the disease.

Pets and Lyme Disease

Ticks can cause problems with pets in two ways. First, ticks can transmit Lyme disease to pets and animals such as cattle, horses, sheep, and rabbits. Second, dogs and cats that go outside may pick up ticks. The pet might bring the ticks indoors, where they may leave the pet and attach to people.

Animals with Lyme disease seldom get a rash. Common symptoms are itching, pain, lack of energy, appetite loss, fever, and swollen joints. Animals may limp or walk or move with difficulty. An animal with any of these symptoms needs to visit a veterinarian right away.

It's important to check pets for ticks once or twice a day in tick areas. Examine pets closely. Ticks like to crawl around the head and inside the ears. Use a comb with fine teeth to remove unattached ticks.

Remove any attached ticks at once in the same way you would remove one from yourself. Put the tick into a plastic bag or container with a cover, seal, and label. The label should include the date, pet name, animal type, and the owner's name, address, and telephone number. Clean the bite site, your hands, and the tweezers. Bring the pet and tick to the vet if possible. With early diagnosis, antibiotics often stop Lyme disease infection.

> **Myth vs. Fact**
>
> **Myth:** People who get Lyme disease once never will get it again.
>
> **Fact:** People who have had Lyme disease aren't immune. They can get Lyme disease again if an infected tick bites them.

Many tick control products are available for pets and livestock. Flea and tick collars can help repel ticks for dogs and cats. Sprays and dips kill ticks on dogs, cats, and horses. Treat outdoor areas for animals with tick control products. Vets may recommend a Lyme disease vaccine for dogs who go outside regularly. The vaccine lasts five to six months. There is no vaccine for animals other than dogs.

Hope for the Future

Early diagnosis and treatment provide the best chance of recovery. Scientists are working to find better tests for diagnosing the disease. They also are working on a vaccine that will cause ticks to die before they can transmit Lyme disease.

Points to Consider

Have you been bitten by a tick? How did you remove it?

Do you have a pet? Do you check your pet regularly for ticks? After reading this chapter, will you check your pet more often for ticks?

What advice would you give to a friend who is going to a Lyme disease area for the first time?

What can you do to educate other people about Lyme disease?

Glossary

acute (uh-KYOOT)—appearing suddenly, increasing rapidly, and getting worse quickly

allergic reaction (a-LUR-jik ree-AK-shuhn)—rejection of and reaction to a drug in the body.

arthritis (arth-RYE-tuhss)—swelling, stiffness, and pain in a joint in the body

chronic (KRON-ik)—continuing for a long time; a person with a chronic disease or illness may have it throughout life.

genitals (JEN-uh-tuhlz)—the sex organs

host (HOHST)—the living animal or person that provides food for ticks; a person, bird or other wild animal, or pet can be a host for ticks.

immune system (i-MYOON SISS-tuhm)—the system that protects the body from illness and disease

joint (JOINT)—a point where movable body parts are connected, such as the knee joint

microorganism (mye-kroh-OR-guh-niz-uhm)—tiny living thing such as bacteria

parasite (PAR-uh-site)—something that feeds off a living animal; parasites get food from the blood and tissue fluid of its host.

relapse (REE-lapss)—the return of symptoms after a period of improvement

repellent (ri-PEL-uhnt)—a substance used to keep ticks away

side effect (SIDE i-FEKT)—an unpleasant or unwanted reaction to a drug

symptom (SIMP-tuhm)—evidence or sign of something, such as an illness

vaccine (vak-SEEN)—a liquid containing weakened or dead bacteria; vaccines cause the body to produce antibodies against a specific disease.

For More Information

Karlen, Arno. *Biography of a Germ*. New York: Pantheon, 2000.

Vanderhoof-Forschner, Karen. *Everything You Need to Know About Lyme Disease and Other Tick-Borne Disorders*. New York: Wiley, 1997.

Veggeberg, Scott. *Lyme Disease*. Springfield, NJ: Enslow, 1998.

Weitzman, Elizabeth. *Let's Talk About Having Lyme Disease*. New York: PowerKids Press, 1997.

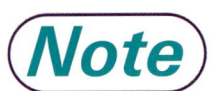

Note: At publication, all resources listed here were accurate and appropriate to the topics covered in this book. Addresses and phone numbers may change. When visiting Internet sites and links, use good judgment. Remember, never give personal information over the Internet.

Useful Addresses and Internet Sites

Arthritis Foundation
1330 West Peachtree Street
Atlanta, Georgia 30309
1-800-283-7800
www.arthritis.org/answers/teens.asp
Information for teens on arthritis

Centers for Disease Control and Prevention
National Center for Infectious Diseases
Division of Vector-Borne Infectious Diseases
PO Box 2087
Fort Collins, CO 80522
www.cdc.gov

Lyme Alliance, Inc.
PO Box 454
Concord, MI 49237
www.lymealliance.org
Articles and resources

Lyme Borreliosis Society
Box 91535
West Vancouver, BC V7V 3P2
CANADA

Lyme Disease Foundation
One Financial Plaza, 18th Floor
Hartford, CT 06103
1-800-886-5963
www.lyme.org
Resources and links

Lyme Disease Network of New Jersey
43 Winton Road
East Brunswick, NJ 08816
www.lymenet.org
Articles on Lyme disease

National Institute of Allergy and
Infectious Diseases (NIAID)
National Institutes of Health
Building 31, Room 7A50
31 Center Drive
MSC 2520
Bethesda, MD 20892-2520
www.niaid.nih.gov/publications/tick.htm
Information and overview of Lyme disease and its treatment

Index

aches, 8, 9, 10, 12, 25, 50. *See also* stiffness
allergies, 39
antibiotics, 34, 35–37
   for pets, 58
   side effects of, 37–39
antibodies, 28, 48
arthritis, 6, 11, 16, 24, 26, 27, 30, 39, 49

bacteria, 7, 10, 17–20, 28–29, 33–36, 38, 48
birds, 7, 17, 19, 47
blood tests, 28–29
Borrelia burgdorferi (Bb), 7, 17, 19–20
brain, 10, 29, 36
breathing difficulties, 10, 11, 39
brush, 18, 44, 49
bushes, 18, 44, 47–48

Centers for Disease Control and Prevention (CDC), 40
chills, 10, 25, 50
chronic Lyme disease, 6, 11, 24, 26, 35–37
cleanliness, 45–46
clothing, 45–46, 47
concentration problems, 11, 26
control products, 59
cramps, 12, 37
cure, 6, 37, 59

deer, 5, 7, 17, 18, 19, 20, 21, 44, 47
deet, 46–47
diagnosis, 23–31
   difficulties in, 26–27, 29, 30
diarrhea, 37, 38
disseminated Lyme disease, 10, 24, 26, 36
dizziness, 10, 30

doctor, when to call, 5, 12, 25, 57

early local Lyme disease, 8–9, 24, 29, 35–36
erythema migrans (EM), 8–9, 27. *See also* rashes

fever, 5, 9, 10, 25, 50
first aid, 53–59

grassy areas, 16, 18, 20, 21, 27, 44, 45, 47

headaches, 8, 9, 10, 23, 25, 30
heart problems, 8, 10, 11, 24, 26, 27, 36, 39, 49

immune system, 28, 34, 38

joints, 5, 6, 8, 25, 29, 30, 39, 50

late Lyme disease. *See* chronic Lyme disease
leaves, 19, 21, 43, 44, 47
lizards, 51
local Lyme disease. *See* early local Lyme disease
Lyme disease
   acquiring, 15–21
   chronic, 6, 11, 24, 26, 35–37
   diagnosing, 11, 23–31
   disseminated, 10, 24, 26, 36
   early local, 8–9, 35–36
   history, 16
   prevention of, 43–51
   spread of, 16–17, 18–19
   stages of, 8–11
   symptoms of, 6, 8–11, 16, 23–27, 30, 58

Index continued

testing for, 5, 21, 24, 27, 28–29, 57
treating, 6, 33–41
what is it?, 5–13
Lyme disease vaccine, 48–49, 59
Lyme ticks, 7, 16–20, 47

memory problems, 11, 26, 34
mice, 7, 16, 17, 19–20, 44, 47–48
mood changes, 26
multiple sclerosis, 30
muscles, 10, 11, 12, 25, 26, 30, 50
myths, 31, 38, 46, 59

nerve damage, 8, 10, 11, 12, 24, 29, 30, 36, 39

organizations, 40–41

pain, 6, 9, 10–12, 25, 29, 34, 39, 50
pets, 5, 7, 17, 53, 58–59
post-Lyme disease syndrome (PLDS), 34
prevention, 43–51
 avoiding tick areas, 43, 44–45
 proper dress, 45–46, 47
 protecting property, 47–48
 repellents, 46–47

rashes, 5, 8, 9, 10, 11, 23, 25, 27, 39, 46. *See also erythema migrans* (EM)
relapse, 33
repellents, 46–47
rock walls, 47

safety, 53–59
showering, 46, 54
shrubs, 18, 44, 45, 47–48

skin problems, 8, 11, 24, 39. *See also rashes*
sleeping problems, 11, 26
spinal tap, 29
stiffness, 6, 11, 23, 25, 30. *See also aches*
stress, 39
support, 39
swelling, 5, 6, 8, 11, 12, 29, 30, 39
symptoms, 5, 6, 8–11, 16, 23–27, 30
 of pets, 58

testing, 57
tests, medical, 5, 12, 24, 27, 28–29, 57
ticks, 6, 7, 12, 13, 15, 16, 17, 18, 19, 21, 50
 avoiding, 43, 44–45
 checking for, 15, 46, 54–55
 Lyme, 7, 16–20, 47
 and pets, 17, 58–59
 removing, 55, 56–57
tiredness, 5, 8, 10, 11, 12, 23, 34
treatment, 33–41
 early, 6, 34
 stages of, 35–36
tremors, 30
tweezers, 55, 56

vaccine for Lyme disease, 48–49, 59
 for dogs, 59
 problems with, 50
vaginitis, 38

weakness, 10, 26
weather, 20
wooded areas, 20, 23, 26, 27, 43, 44, 49